The Coconut Oil Secret

Why This Tropical Treasure is
Nature's #1 Best Healing Superfood

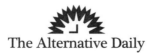

The Alternative Daily

Table of Contents

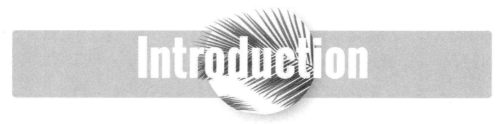

Introduction

One thing is for sure: coconut oil is no fad. For thousands of years, people living in the tropics have used coconut meat, milk, juice and oil for food and medicinal purposes. Spanish explorers called this wonderful health-promoting nut "monkey face," for the three indents on its front that resemble a monkey's face.

Its scientific name is *Cocos nucifera*, meaning "nut-bearing." Coconuts have a long and respected history throughout numerous

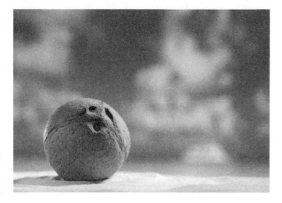

cultures in the world, and many depend on them for their survival. Pacific islanders refer to coconut oil as a cure for all illnesses and many call it the "healthiest oil on earth."

The Alternative Daily

The coconut palm, which produces the coconut, is known as the "Tree of Life," and although many people have been aware of this nut's amazing nutritional quality, they may not know that it is a "functional food."

Functional foods are those that are not only high in vitamins, minerals and fiber, but also possess healing properties. Modern medicine and science are finally catching up with tradition and uncovering the real story behind the coconut and why everyone should use it. As a result of increasing research, many people are responding and starting to replace other oils in their home with coconut oil—this is good news.

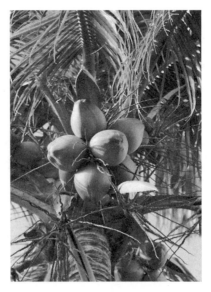

This book is meant to help you better understand how coconut oil can play an integral role in health. Man creates nothing new, he simply repurposes everything he finds in nature - and nothing concocted in a laboratory can ever replace the value of what is found in nature. Seem too simple?

Read on to see how modern science has unlocked the mystery of the fruit of the "Tree of Life."

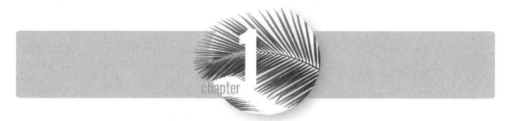

A Brief History

With obesity, heart disease, cancer and diabetes at epidemic proportions, it is time for a new approach that isn't really new after all!

Before World War II, and for about thirty years after, people in such countries as the Philippines consumed a diet of rice, coconuts, vegetables and root crops. They were rarely sick and you had to look really hard to find anyone who was overweight. Conditions such as diabetes, cancer and heart disease were virtually unheard of. People who did visit a doctor did so to have wounds treated or to receive help for tropical diseases such as malaria or dengue

The Alternative Daily

Today most of the world's coconut production comes from small farms in Asia. The crop is easy to grow even in difficult environments and can take poor soil and drought. It also plays a very important role in maintaining the fragile ecosystem of island and coastal regions. Over 70 percent of coconut crops are consumed locally as food, drink and cooking oil. Fibers are fashioned into rope and twine, husks are used for flooring material, shells are made into bowls, utensils and jewelry, leaves become brooms, baskets and mats, and trunks are fashioned into furniture or even homes. In fact, all parts of the tree and coconut are useful in some way or another.

fever. Coconut oil, meat and milk were consumed daily and meals were high in saturated fat from the coconut. The oil was often made by hand through a process of fermentation or boiling.

Not only were coconuts an integral part of traditional diets, they were also used in medicine. Health problems such as coughs, constipation, jaundice, lice, malnutrition, bruises, burns, colds, skin infections, typhoid, toothaches, wounds, scabies, gingivitis, earaches, fevers and flus were often treated using coconuts, especially coconut oil.

With dramatic changes in the way food was processed after World War II, things began to unravel. Sadly, Western food made its way to the tropical cultures and health began to decline. Many of the traditional methods of preparing food, including coconut oil, were replaced by modern, mechanical processes. Large coconut refineries were built to supply the United States with the oil (which was used in the baking industry). Although some people still made their coconut oil by hand, many opted for the cheaper (refined) product that was readily available in the marketplace.

Coconut oil was in demand in America for some time after the war, however, this too ended as the oil was quickly replaced with unhealthy, hydrogenated oils. Many people in countries such as the Philippines were forced to leave their coconut farms behind and move into cities in search of jobs. In addition to this, people began to adopt Western-style diets. Cheaper, mass-produced food replaced local traditional fare and few people cultivated their own food. Fast foods, including those made with highly-refined coconut oil, rice grown with chemical fertilizers, and soft drinks loaded with sugar were consumed in abundance. Obesity became more prevalent, as did Western diseases such as heart disease, diabetes and cancer.

Fortunately, over the last decade, more research is being uncovered revealing the incredible health benefits of unrefined coconut oil. As the volume of research continues to amplify, people all over the world are accepting what Asian and Pacific islanders have known for thousands of years: coconut oil is a delicious, nutritious superfood with medicinal characteristics that should not be ignored.

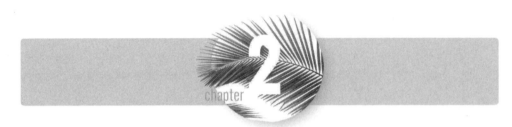

chapter 2

The Saturated Fat Myth

The theory that took saturated fats down, including tropical saturated fat found in coconuts, appeared in the 1950s and has been coined the "lipid hypothesis." This hypothesis stated that there was an intimate relationship between saturated fat, cholesterol and heart disease.

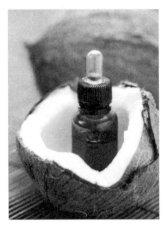

This hypothesis was built on questionable evidence at best. Ancel Keys, the founder of the hypothesis, presented his "findings" to the medical community. Despite a lack of evidence and the prevalence of other studies finding different conclusions, the lipid hypothesis took hold.

The majority of support came from food manufacturers and vegetable oil producers who saw great benefit in promoting this hypothesis. If everyone would stop using saturated fat, they could convince consumers that refined vegetable oil was healthy.

The truth is, almost 90 percent of all well-researched studies examining this hypothesis do not support the fact that saturated fats and dietary cholesterol cause heart disease. In fact, researchers have found that a clogged artery is composed of about 26 percent saturated fat and more than half polyunsaturated fat.

Since the 1960s, there have been a wealth of studies assuring us that saturated fats found in dairy products, such as butter and whole milk, as well as red meats, increase "bad" LDL cholesterol levels and contribute to heart disease.

These studies spearheaded our nation's obsession with "low-fat" products, and a campaign began promoting the use of polyunsaturated fats such as corn, safflower and soybean oil.

The Lipid Hypothesis Just Doesn't Make Sense

Although you will find a number of studies where researchers have induced heart disease in animals by loading them up with huge doses of oxidized and rancid cholesterol (about 10 times the amount found in the ordinary human diet), modern research contradicts the cholesterol-heart disease connection.

The Alternative Daily

Famous heart surgeon Michael E. DeBakey found that in a survey of 1,700 patients with hardening of the arteries, there was no relationship at all between the level of cholesterol in the blood and the predominance of atherosclerosis.

A study of adults in South Carolina found no relationship between blood cholesterol levels and the consumption of red meat, animal fat, butter, eggs, bacon, sausage, cheese or whole milk. On the contrary, a survey conducted by the Medical Research Council showed that men who ate butter had half the risk of developing heart disease than those men who consumed margarine.

Residents of northern India eat 17 times more animal fat than those in southern India. However, they have a seven times lower rate of heart disease. Eskimos eat a lot of saturated fat from fish and other animals but they are virtually free from disease.

The French are another example of a group of people who consume large amounts of saturated fats from butter, eggs, cheese, cream, liver and other meats but have a much lower rate of coronary heart disease than many other countries in the West. In the United States, 315 of every 100,000 middle-aged men die of heart attacks each year; in France the rate is 145 per 100,000.

Avoid Trans Fats

One thing is certain: the type of fat that should be avoided the most is trans fat, also known as partially hydrogenated oil. Often included in so-called "low fat" foods, this fake fat is highly dangerous. The main sources of trans fats are processed, baked goods and fast foods.

These types of fats raise levels of "bad" LDL cholesterol, while reducing levels of "good" HDL cholesterol. It is best to stay away from trans fats altogether, they offer absolutely no health benefits.

The inflammatory properties of these oils observed by some studies may well be due to the methods used in processing and packaging these oils, and not a property of the oils themselves.

The more natural a fat source is, and the less processing involved in its creation, the healthier it usually is. There are exceptions, such as the hormone-disrupting dangers of soybean oil. However, aside from these known "risk-factor foods," when you choose natural, it is hard to go wrong.

TRUTH: It is also important to understand that early coconut research was conducted on highly refined coconut oil that contained dangerous trans fats.

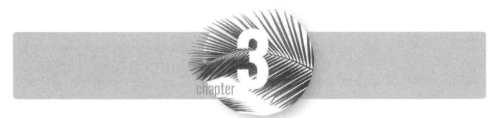

Types of Coconut Oil

Like most things, not all coconut oil is created equal; some are better than others. Obviously, the more processed the oil is, the less health benefits it possesses. But, let's take a closer look at just what is the best type of coconut oil to purchase if you are seeking optimal therapeutic and nutritional value.

Less than 15 years ago, coconut oil was rare on shelves in America, today this is not the case. There are many types and brands to choose from and like other things, this can become confusing. Knowing which type of coconut oil to purchase can be the difference when seeking to reap its potent therapeutic value.

Although there may be a lot of terminology used, there really are only two broad types of coconut oil. One is heavily processed and one is minimally processed. We say, minimally processed because coconut oil - unlike an apple or a banana - does not have a totally pure and unrefined form delivered directly from nature. Although coconuts do grow on trees - the oil does not. All oil has to somehow be extracted from the whole coconut. The only truly unprocessed and unrefined coconut oil you can consume is that which is still in the meat that comes directly from the coconut just picked off of the tree.

What is Copra?

Copra is the termed used by industry leaders in coconut products (mainly the Philippines) and refers to dried coconut that has been removed from the shell. To dry the coconut, any number of methods may be used including smoke drying, kiln drying, sun drying - or any combination of these. After drying, the coconut is inedible and requires more processing. The product is only good for industrial use at this point. Copra has its own place in the market and is exported to the United States where it is further refined for industrial use only.

The Alternative Daily

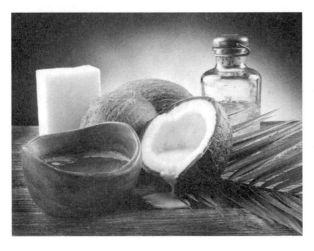

Choosing the Best Coconut Oil

When you visit your local grocer or health food store or are surfing your way around the Internet, you may see any number of terms used to describe coconut oil. So, how do you know which is best? Here are just a few tips to help you make the best choice possible.

Refined coconut oil: Although the term sounds insanely industrial, refined coconut oil is edible. In fact, this form of coconut oil is the type of dietary oil that is used by millions of people in tropical countries.

Refined coconut oils are generally referred to as RBD coconut oils. The acronym simply stands for: Refined, Bleached, Deodorized. Bleaching is generally not a chemical process like one would think but rather a filtration process using a bleaching clay that is used to remove impurities. Steam is used to deodorize the oil.

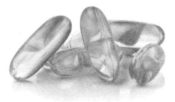

This coconut oil will no longer have that distinctive tropical smell that we are familiar with. Manufacturers add chemicals such as sodium hydroxide in order to prolong the shelf life.

This method of processing does not alter the fatty acid content of the coconut oil, however, it does strip away nutrients.

Types of Refined Coconut Oils

Expeller pressed coconut oil - this coconut oil is produced using physical refining processes, not chemical. It is generally thought to be cleaner than oil that is refined with solvent extracts such as hexane.

Coconut oil (no other descriptor) - if the label does not indicate any particular type of coconut oil - it is most likely RBD coconut oil. You need to be careful with this type of coconut oil because it could be made from copra that has been chemically refined - generally processed with dangerous solvents.

Liquid coconut oil - In 2013 a new name for coconut oil appeared. Liquid coconut oil is not, however, a new product. This oil that stays liquid even in the refrigerator, is actually fractionated coconut oil - or oil that has had lauric acid removed. Also known as MCT oil - it is used mostly in skin care products, but lately has been marketed as a dietary supplement. Be careful with this - MCT oil is actually a by-product of the lauric acid industry. Although it is a versatile oil because it is not solid - it is highly processed and does not contain the beneficial ingredient, lauric acid.

Hydrogenated coconut oil - Run fast from this coconut oil - it contains dangerous trans fats. Although it keeps solid at higher temperatures, this is no trade off for the health dangers it poses. Although you may not see this product in the store as a coconut oil - it may be used in the processed food industry. If you see the term "hydrogenated coconut oil" as an ingredient in any product - don't buy it!

Virgin coconut oil: The least processed of all coconut oil is known as virgin. The term "virgin coconut oil" was used starting around 2000 as a means to differentiate between the least refined coconut oil and the more readily available refined coconut oil on the market.

Virgin coconut oil can be made one of two ways - either by pressing the oil out of the dried coconut or by a process known as wet-milling.

Dried Process:

Fresh coconut meat is dried first and later the oil is pressed out. This is higher grade coconut oil than the RBD type as the process starts with fresh coconut not the copra.

Wet-Milling:

During the wet-milling process, oil is pressed out of a wet emulsion or "coconut milk". The oil is then separated from water by any number of methods including boiling, fermentation, refrigeration, enzymes or the use of a mechanical centrifuge.

Several studies show that fermentation, which uses heat, yields the coconut oil with the highest amount of antioxidants. During this process freshly grated coconut is used to make a coconut milk emulsion. Heavy water sinks to the bottom of the container and the oil stays on the top along with some other coconut solids. The oil is taken out and put in a large wok and heated until the solids sink to the bottom of the pan. The oil is then filtered. Keep in mind that because coconut oil is stable at relatively high heat - the heating of the oil in this process does not damage the oil in any way.

What about extra virgin coconut oil

So, if we know that virgin coconut oil is good for us, is extra virgin even better? In reality, there is no difference between extra virgin and virgin coconut oils. This is simply a marketing term, nothing else.

The Alternative Daily

What about GMO coconut oil?

There is no genetically modified coconut oil - and very few pests that trouble coconut trees. If any pesticides are used, they do not impact the coconut themselves because they grow so high up in the trees.

What about organic coconut oil?

The organic certification of coconut oil is very costly and few actually have this label. As long as you know that the coconut oil was processed through traditional fermentation methods - it is not essential to purchase organic. Certified organic coconut oil can be made out of organic dried coconut - not necessarily using the wet-milling process that yields higher antioxidants.

Hands down, at the end of the day the best coconut oil is made from a wet-milling process using fermentation/heating.

Properties of Coconut Oil

- **Antibacterial**—stops bacteria that cause gum disease, throat infections, urinary tract infections and ulcers in their tracks.

- **Anticarcinogenic**—keeps dangerous cancer cells from spreading while boosting immunity.

- **Antifungal**—destroys infection-promoting fungus and yeast.

- **Anti-inflammatory**—suppresses inflammation and repairs tissue.

- **Antimicrobial**—inactivates harmful microbes and fights infection.

The Alternative Daily

- **Antioxidant**—protects from free radical damage.

- **Antiretroviral**—destroys HIV and HTLV-1.

- **Antiparasitic**—rids the body of lice, tapeworms and other parasites.

- **Anti-protozoa**—kills protozoan infection in the gut.

- **Antiviral**—kills viruses that cause influenza, herpes, measles, AIDS, hepatitis and more.

- **Improves nutrient absorption**—really easy to digest and makes nutrients readily available.

- **Safe and nontoxic**

- **No side effects**

Lauric, Capric and Caprylic Acid

Half of the fat in coconut oil is comprised of a fat that is not frequently found in nature, lauric acid. Lauric acid has been called a "miracle" ingredient due to its health promoting capabilities, and is present in a mother's milk. In fact, it can be found in only three dietary sources—small amounts in butterfat and larger amounts in palm kernel and coconut oils.

In the body, lauric acid is converted to monolaurin, which is a potent antiviral, antibacterial and antiprotozoal substance. Because monolaurin is a monoglyceride, it can destroy lipid-coated viruses including measles, influenza, HIV, herpes and a number of pathogenic bacteria.

> ## Coconut oil contains the most lauric acid of any substance on Earth!

Coconut oil also contains another fatty acid, capric acid. Capric acid is present in very small amounts in goat's milk and cow's milk, but is abundant in tropical oils including coconut oil and palm kernel oil. It is a medium-chain fatty acid that has potent antimicrobial and antiviral properties. In the body, capric acid is converted to monocaprin, a form that can readily fight viruses, bacteria and the yeast Candida albicans.

The third fatty acid that coconut oil contains is caprylic acid. This fat is found in mother's breast milk and coconuts. Also known as octanoic acid, this saturated fatty acid has a number of health promoting properties. The Health and Science Institute tells us that caprylic acid has the innate ability to treat yeast-like fungus in the intestines. This makes it great ammunition against Candida (more to come). The Physicians' Desk Reference for Nutritional

Supplements tells us that caprylic acid may also help those who suffer from Crohn's disease, and may have a beneficial impact on high blood pressure. A Japanese study found that caprylic acid suppresses the secretion of IL-8, the gene present in the intestines of those suffering from Crohn's disease.

Daily Supplementation Dosage

Although coconut oil is safe, you should check with a health professional for the correct dosage.

Weight	Amount
Above 175 pounds	4 tbsp.
Above 150 pounds	3.5 tbsp.
Above 125 pounds	3 tbsp.
Above 100 pounds	2.5 tbsp.
Above 75 pounds	1.5 tbsp.
Above 50 pounds	1.5 tsp.
Above 25 pounds	1 tsp.

One great way to get your daily dose of coconut oil is to switch out other oils with coconut oil. Coconut oil can be substituted equally for any oil for cooking and also used as a replacement for butter if desired.

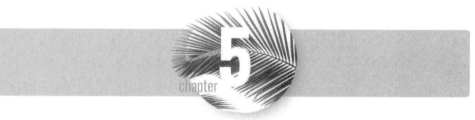

A Quick Look at Chemistry

Ninety-two percent of the fat found in coconut oil is saturated. Compare this to olive oil, which is 15 percent saturated, beef fat, which is 50 percent saturated and butter, which is 63 percent saturated. The fact that the oil is so high in saturated fat explains why it remains solid at room temperature and does not go rancid quickly. Many vegans use it as a butter substitute.

Besides its high saturated fat content, coconut oil also contains a high number of medium-chain triglycerides (or medium-chain fatty acids, known as MCTs), which contain 6-12 carbons (more on MCTs to come).

In fact, coconut oil is the richest source of these medium-chain fatty acids. This is compared to most other oils, which are made up of long-chain triglycerides (LCTs) and have more than 12 carbons. Soybean oil is 100 percent LCTs and coconut oil has 40 percent LCTs and 60 percent MCTs. This makes a huge difference because of the way our bodies metabolize MCTs and LCTs.

LCTs are very difficult for the body to break down and require a special enzyme for digestion. They also put a great deal of strain on the pancreas, liver and digestive system. The body stores LCTs primarily as fat, and they are also deposited into arteries in lipid forms such as cholesterol.

In stark contrast, MCTs have numerous health promoting qualities. They are much smaller than LCTs, which means they can permeate cell membranes easily and do not require special enzymes to be functional to the body. They are easy to digest and are also sent directly to the liver where they are converted to energy—not stored as fat. MCTs also help to stimulate metabolism.

Coconut Oil Fuels the Fat Burning Furnace

As use of traditional animal and tropical oils has decreased, the waistlines and preponderance of diseases, such as heart disease, cancer and hypercholesterolemia, have increased. There has even been a marked increase in the number of obese children due to widespread use of hydrogenated oils in fast and processed foods.

Researchers have discovered that in cultures where unrefined coconut oil is a part of the everyday diet, there is less obesity and less lifestyle-related disease. As was mentioned earlier, the shorter-chain fatty acids found in coconut oil burn quickly in the body.

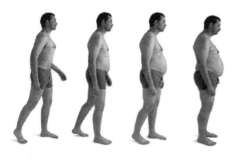

They are like small pieces of dry kindling added to a fire as opposed to a big damp log. The immediate transport of MCTs to the liver means the fat does not have to be transported through the whole body first and does not end up as fat in the blood, but remains accessible fat that can be used to power the body.

MCTs also increase the rate at which the body burns fuel for energy. When you look at the lean and trim bodies of people living in the tropics—who make coconut a staple in their diets—this makes a lot of sense.

"During the past 20 years, there has been a dramatic increase in obesity in the United States and rates remain high. In 2010, no state had a prevalence of obesity less than 20%. Thirty-six states had a prevalence of 25% or more; 12 of these states (Alabama, Arkansas, Kentucky, Louisiana, Michigan, Mississippi, Missouri, Oklahoma, South Carolina, Tennessee, Texas, and West Virginia) had a prevalence of 30% or more."—
US Centers for Disease Control

A well-known population study conducted in the South Pacific islands of Pukapuka and Tokelau, located close to New Zealand, began in the 1960s before the areas had been exposed to refined foods from the West. People living in these areas ate only traditional foods and coconut was consumed at each meal in one way or another.

For these islanders, 50 to 60 percent of their calories came from fat, most in the form of saturated fat from coconuts. In comparison people living in the West were getting about 30 to 40 percent of calories from fat. Compared to Western standards, the health of both island populations was very good. They had no sign of kidney disease, hypothyroidism or high blood cholesterol. All of the people were lean and very healthy with ideal height to weight ratios. Western diseases such as heart disease, colitis, colon cancer, ulcers, atherosclerosis and appendicitis were very rare.

This is not the only study conducted on the effects of diets high in saturated fat. In the 1930s, a dentist, Dr. Weston Price, conducted studies on people living in the Pacific islands. He was very interested in how traditional diets influenced overall health and well-being, specifically dental health. He compared populations of islanders who ate traditional food with those who ate refined food. Dr. Price discovered that islanders who ate traditional fare were in great health and not overweight despite the fact that they ate large amounts of saturated fat. Those who traded food with Western countries and ate a higher percentage of refined foods (high in carbohydrates) suffered from common Western diseases including obesity and tooth decay.

The Indian Department of Medicine conducted a study comparing traditional cooking oils and fats, such as clarified butter and coconut oil, which are high in saturated fats, with oils such as safflower and sunflower, which are mostly polyunsaturated fats. Use of these oils was compared to incidences of type 2 diabetes and heart disease.

What was discovered was that as saturated fats were replaced with polyunsaturated fats, the rates of heart disease and diabetes went up. The so-called "heart friendly" oils contain a bad ratio of omega-6 fatty acids to omega-3 fatty acids. Additional studies have indicated that consumption of modern vegetable oils can harm one's health.

A random, double-blind study divided women into two groups: one group received soybean oil supplements (S) and the other group (C) received the same amount of virgin coconut oil. Each group was instructed to follow a balanced diet and walk 50 minutes each day.

The results:

"[After one week,] only group C exhibited a reduction in [waist circumference]... Group S presented an increase... in total cholesterol, LDL and LDL:HDL ratio, whilst HDL diminished... Such alterations were not observed in group C. It appears that dietetic supplementation with coconut oil does not cause dyslipidemia and seems to promote a reduction in abdominal obesity."

Similar findings were revealed in a 2003 study. It was found that consumption of MCTs increased energy expenditure and reduced adipose fat in overweight men. When 24 overweight men consumed diets rich in MCTs or LCTs, the group consuming MCTs lost more weight and had an increase in energy compared to those consuming LCTs.

A study of 40 women with abdominal obesity consumed 1 ounce of coconut oil per day and had a significant reduction of BMI and waist circumference in 12 weeks. In another study, 20 obese males had a 1.1 inch reduction in waist size after only 4 weeks of consuming 1 ounce of coconut oil per day.

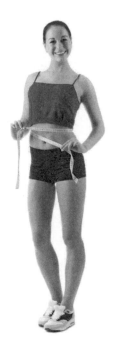

Feel Full Longer

Coconut oil can also reduce hunger. One study found that men who ate the most MCTs consumed 256 fewer calories than men who did not. In another study, men who had MCTs for breakfast ate far fewer calories throughout the day than men who did not eat MCTs.

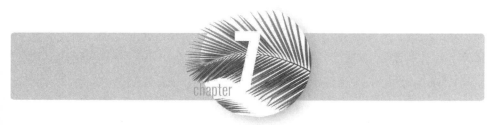

chapter 7

Boosting Your Thyroid

Over 13 million people in America suffer from low thyroid function. There is strong reason to believe that an underactive thyroid is a major block to weight loss, especially for women. Thyroid hormones are necessary for normal health and cellular activity and if thyroid function is not normal, weight loss is next to impossible.

The thyroid gland is responsible for controlling the temperature of the body, and use of energy and growth rate in children. Fatigue, depression, weight gain, cold hands and feet, sensitivity to cold, low body temperature, headaches, joint pain, menstrual disorders, puffy eyes, hair loss, brittle nails, constipation, ringing in the ears, loss of sex drive and frequent infections are all possible indicators of a sluggish thyroid.

It is thought that diet plays a role in thyroid health. Although low iodine intake leads to low thyroid function, table salt does not appear to be the best option. Many foods eaten in Western culture contain what are known as goitrogens or iodine blockers. Two popular goitrogens are soybeans and peanuts. A great amount of processed foods contain either or both of these. Grocery store items are full of polyunsaturated oils and many Americans still shy away from using saturated fat, preferring to cook with expeller-pressed or solvent-extracted oils. If you cook with vegetable oil, it is time to stop.

Polyunsaturated oils such as soy oil have been used to fatten up livestock. These oils, comprised of LCTs, promote weight gain. In the 1940s farmers tried using coconut oil to fatten animals and discovered that it made them lean and active instead.

With the industrialization of our agricultural system, soil has become iodine deficient, further compromising thyroid health. In addition, consumption of refined sugars and grains also negatively impact thyroid function. There are also a number of environmental stressors such as chemical pollutants, pesticides, mercury and fluoride that stress the thyroid. With all these insults, it is no wonder so many people suffer from inadequate thyroid function.

A Note about Rancidity

Vegetable oils oxidize very rapidly and become rancid. To prevent rancidity, food manufacturers super-refine the oils, which is especially damaging to cell health and causes a negative impact on the thyroid. The long-chain fatty acids found in vegetable oils that are deposited in cells are often rancid, oxidized fat, which interferes with the conversion of the thyroid hormone T4 to T3, needed to produce enzymes for the conversion of fat to energy.

Coconut Oil to the Rescue

Because coconut oil is saturated and highly stable, oxidation does not occur, and because it is broken down differently in the body, coconut oil does not interfere with the conversion of T4 to T3. In addition to changing from polyunsaturated fats to healthy saturated fats found in coconut oil, there are a number of other healthy lifestyle changes you can make to support healthy thyroid function:

- Consume iodine-rich foods such as sea vegetables, cranberries, freshly caught fish and eggs.

- Juice organic vegetables.

- Avoid foods that contain soybean oil—often found in mayonnaise, peanut butter, dressings, etc..

- Reduce consumption of processed grains and sugar.

- Limit exposure to fluoride and mercury—have a good water-filtration system for your home.

- Take high-quality supplements such as zinc, selenium, manganese, chromium, B vitamins, vitamin C, vitamin A and vitamin E (Cod liver oil is a good source of natural vitamin A).

- Exercise—this is especially important to correct thyroid function. Walking briskly for 30 minutes a day is a good place to start.

These studies, and more, make a strong case for virgin coconut oil. If you want to feed your metabolic furnace, improve your energy and drop belly fat, add virgin coconut oil to a well-balanced healthy daily diet. MCT oil is an easy substitution in salad dressings, smoothies and soups.

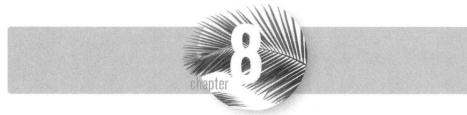

Brain Health

According to the Alzheimer's Association, the number of people diagnosed with this debilitating disease is on the rise. It is expected that by the year 2050, almost 14 million people will be living with the condition known to rob people of their memories and impose anxiety and confusion.

Presently, over 5 million people suffer the effects of this disease that is now known as the 7th leading cause of death in our country. It is estimated that over 148 billion dollars are spent each year treating Alzheimer's.

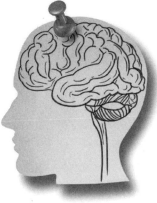

The Alternative Daily

There are no pharmaceutical options available to treat, halt or reverse the symptoms of Alzheimer's disease. Drugs being created now are made to reduce the amyloid plaques, made from a protein called Amyloid B (AB), that build up on the brain. These are a trademark of the disease.

However, recent studies reveal that small clumps of AB, called oligomers, appear years before the plaques even start to develop. The molecular structure of these oligomers is very different from AB.

Further, they found that drugs designed to destroy amyloid plaques have no effect on oligomers. This could explain why experimental Alzheimer's drugs have failed; they are focused on plaques, not their precursor, oligomers.

Case Study: A Natural Approach

Mary Newport, MD, has had some up-close and highly personal experience with dementia and Alzheimer's. When her 53-year-old husband started showing signs of progressive dementia, which was later diagnosed as Alzheimer's, she took action.

He began taking Alzheimer's drugs such as Namenda, Exelon and Aricept—however, his disease continued to worsen. It was not until Dr. Newport tried to get her husband into a drug trial for a new Alzheimer's drug that she started to research Alzheimer's triggers.

Her research led her to the discovery that some brain cells may have a difficult time using glucose—the brain's main source of energy. Without this fuel, neurons begin to die. An alternative energy source for brain cells is fats, known as ketones. When the body is deprived of carbohydrates, it naturally produces ketones.

The hard part is that most people can't cut carbohydrates out of the body altogether, and in many respects this can be unhealthy. So another way to produce ketones is by consuming oils made from medium-chain triglycerides. MCT is an oil made from coconut and palm oil.

The drug being used in the trial was just MCT oil at a dose of 20 grams. When MCT oil is metabolized, ketones, which are created by the body, not only protect against Alzheimer's but may also reverse the symptoms. This is also a potential treatment for Parkinson's, Huntington's, type 2 diabetes, multiple sclerosis and amyotrophic lateral sclerosis (ALS or Lou Gehrig's disease).

Mr. Newport began to take coconut oil twice a day at a point where he could not even remember how to draw a clock. After taking two tablespoons of virgin coconut oil, he had an immediate increase in brain function.

The Alternative Daily

Two weeks after adding coconut oil to his diet, his drawing ability improved. After a little over a month, the drawing had more clarity. It appeared as though the oil was lifting the fog.

After sixty days, he was alert, talkative and happy. He had more focus and concentration and was able to stay on task. He kept taking the same amount of coconut oil each day and the dementia continued to reverse.

He was able to run again, and his reading comprehension improved dramatically. Over time, his short-term memory returned, and he was able to talk about past events with clarity. When he had a brain scan, the atrophy that had once been present was halted.

What We Know

We know that Alzheimer's drugs have failed. We know that a drug company put a non-patentable natural substance (MCT) through an FDA trial, and it worked. But, it has now been discovered that a natural substance can be substituted for an expensive drug.

The amazing thing is that the natural substitute works better than the drug version. The ketones actually last for eight hours in the body when coconut oil is used versus three when the synthetic version is used. If this actually catches on, it could bring the drug monopolies to their knees!

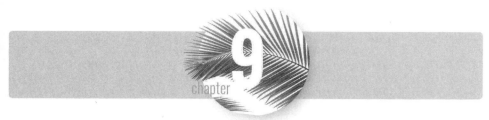

Coconut Oil and Detoxification

Just a quick search on the Internet reveals the popularity of detoxes. Although many of the detoxes touted on the Internet are built around fads and are not scientifically grounded, a true and safe detox has many health promoting benefits:

- Elimination of bacteria

- Improved digestion

- Enhanced immunity

- Improved energy

- Increased metabolism

The Alternative Daily

The key to a successful detox is choosing the right detox method. There is no shortage of options from juicing to full week retreats. However, you don't need to break the bank in order to successfully cleanse.

Coconut oil contains many healing properties that are an integral part of a number of very popular detox programs. In some programs, coconut oil is used as a food replacement. The idea is that every time you are hungry, you take two tablespoons of coconut oil. Since it is easy to digest and provides immediate energy, it is a great substitute for a heavy meal. If you plan on using coconut oil in this manner, it is always best to contact a health professional before beginning. Other popular detoxes combine coconut oil and juicing. The MCTs in the oil act like a carbohydrate in the body, providing an immediate energy boost without spiking insulin. No matter what type of detox you choose, coconut oil is an excellent complement that will keep you energized and feeling full.

Oil Pulling

Oil pulling is a highly powerful way to detoxify the body. Dr. Bruce Fife is a coconut oil expert and the author of *Oil Pulling Therapy*. He says, "oil pulling is one of the most remarkable methods of detoxi-fication and healing I have ever experienced in my career as a naturopathic physician." This process removes bacteria, toxins and parasites from the mouth and also loosens sinuses and congestion while encouraging the lymph system to move toxins out of the body.

Oil Pulling Instructions:

1. Oil pulling should be done on an empty stomach first thing in the morning.

2. Use one tablespoon of organic virgin coconut oil—you may want to start with 1/2 a tablespoon and work your way up to a tablespoon.

3. Swish the oil around your mouth slowly and be sure that the oil reaches all parts of your mouth—do not swallow.

4. Swish for ten minutes minimum.

5. Spit out when you are done and rinse with pure water.

6. Brush with a natural toothpaste afterwards.

7. Oil pulling can be done daily and will reduce plaque, whiten teeth, freshen breath and improve overall health and well-being.

The Alternative Daily

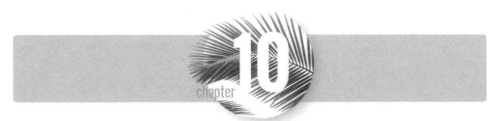

A Word about Cholesterol and Statins

Today, over 40 million people worldwide take prescription statins to lower their levels of LDL cholesterol. However, in doing so, important cellular functions are severely compromised.

HDL and LDL cholesterols serve as carriers of essential CoQ10, beta carotene, and vitamin E to the mitochondria, the energy source of cells. CoQ10 is essential to the functioning of heart muscles, and cholesterol itself is vital for the body's overall function, including brain function and hormonal stability.

Cholesterol Blocking Artery

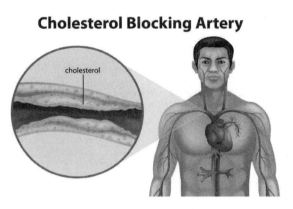

When cholesterol is prevented from doing its job, the body is not able to work as it should. Numerous statin patients testify that they developed a number of new health conditions when they started taking statins, which gradually improved when statin use was stopped.

Some of the most common were severe memory impairment, loss of energy, depression, muscle pain and eye problems. Researchers estimate that only about 1 in 200 adverse effects of statins are actually reported by physicians.

One of the most frightening facts about statins is that in 75 percent of cases, they are prescribed to healthy individuals for preventative purposes, as a "primary prevention" measure against heart disease. However, overwhelming research shows that using statins for primary prevention does nothing to increase life expectancy.

Studies show that the instances of heart attacks in statin patients were somewhat lower, but this was cancelled out by the other diseases that occurred in these patients while on statins, very likely caused by the statins themselves due to their inhibition of cellular function and their blockage of vital nutrients.

In the 25 percent of patients prescribed statins after a cardiac event, stroke, or surgical heart intervention, the statins did increase life expectancy slightly. However, when the statistics were compiled, the life expectancy of these patients rose by only 14 days.

Statins are one of the most widely prescribed classes of drugs in the world, and provide the pharmaceutical industry with billions of dollars in profits each year. Dr. John Abramson of Harvard Medical School explains how the scientific evidence backing statin use is entirely influenced by commercial interests.

In an interview, he details how starting in the Reagan administration, government funding for research in the public interest was significantly cut, and how the great majority of funding for research now comes from the drug companies themselves.

"You have five times better odds of getting the results you want if you pay for the science," Dr. Abramson states. "The real data is not available to the editors of the journal or the peer reviewers."

One example of how the pharmaceutical companies with commercial interest in statins doctored studies supporting their use is the JUPITER Trial. Several years ago, this extremely popular study presented that statins reduce the risk of heart attacks by 54 percent, causing doctors worldwide to prescribe them in huge numbers.

However, Dr. Abramson explains that this was a "relative percentage," and when the actual numbers were analyzed, it was discovered that heart attacks were only reduced by 0.48 percent.

Nethertheless, the media took the JUPITER Trial as fact, and widely reported the success of statins. According to Dr. Abramson, "the only media in the United States that got it right was that renowned medical expert Dr. Stephen Colbert, who said, 'the JUPITER Trial was a great breakthrough in figuring out how to get people to take drugs who don't need them.'"

Heart disease is a serious problem worldwide, causing 7.8 million deaths in 2008. As the death toll continues to rise, it is no surprise that people are afraid and wish to take preventative measures.

However, increasing evidence shows that lowering cholesterol is not the answer, and the use of statins causes great harm with very questionable benefits, at best. The documentary Statin Nation proposes a strong link between stress levels and heart disease, a link that demands further study, as it may hold the key to saving a great number of lives.

Dr. Abramson puts it bluntly: "Hopefully when we look back on this era, and we see the fraud that went on in misleading physicians about the scientific evidence, we'll see that this stands as organized crime… of a higher tech nature than robbing banks with machine guns. But there's a lot more money in this, and in fact, many, many more people get hurt."

Dr. Natasha Campbell-McBride agrees. She urges us to rethink our obsession with cholesterol. "The last thing you want to do is interfere with your blood levels of cholesterol. Your body knows what it is doing. Whatever level of cholesterol you have in your blood at that moment is the right level for you. Don't mess around with it."

Coconut Oil and Cholesterol Profile

The saturated fat in coconut oil can actually protect you from suffering a heart attack or a stroke. Including unrefined coconut oil in the diet generally increases HDL cholesterol and improves the overall cholesterol profile. One of the best indicators of heart disease risk is not to assess total cholesterol, but rather the LDL/HDL ratio. Since coconut oil increases HDL, the overall cholesterol ratio improves, lowering the risk of heart disease.

Research shows that people who consume large amounts of coconut oil as part of their ordinary diet have very low incidences of heart disease and normal cholesterol profiles. The medium-chain fatty acids in coconut oil appear to be what protects the heart. Studies back as far as 1970 demonstrate that coconut oil is heart-friendly, even though it is a saturated fat. In addition to improving the cholesterol profile, consumption of coconut oil lowers body deposition, reduces blood clots, reduces free radicals in cells, and lowers the levels of cholesterol in the blood and liver while increasing the antioxidant reserves in cells. This along with population studies indicating a lower incidence of heart disease demonstrates the effectiveness of coconut oil to protect the heart.

Heart Disease and Infection

Hardening of the arteries (atherosclerosis) causes heart disease. The current thinking on atherosclerosis is that it develops as a result of an injury to the inner lining of the arterial wall. A number of things can cause the injury, such as toxins, free radicals, bacteria and viruses. If the root of the damage is not dealt with, irritation and inflammation will persist and scar tissue will continue to form.

Platelets, which are special blood-clotting proteins, circulate in the blood and when they find an injury, they become sticky and adhere to each other as well as to the damaged tissue, acting like a Band-Aid. This is how a blood clot is formed. Injury of any kind causes platelets to clot together and to release protein growth factors, which encourage the muscle cells in the artery walls to grow. Scar tissue, calcium, platelets, cholesterol and triglycerides rush to the site in an effort to heal the injured area. This results in a mass of arterial plaque. When this plaque builds up in the coronary artery (which feeds the heart) it is called coronary heart disease—the most common cause of death in the United States.

There is also convincing evidence that chronic low-grade infection appears to encourage the development of plaque that leads to heart disease. A Finnish study found that 27 out of 40 heart attack patients and 15 out of 30 men with heart disease carried antibodies that related to chlamydia, which is known to cause gum disease and lung infections. Only seven out of 41 men who were free of heart disease had the antibodies. In an animal study where rabbits were infected with chlamydia, the arterial walls of the rabbits were thickened. Once the rabbits were given an antibiotic the walls reduced to normal size.

A chronic infection may persist without any visible symptoms. It may be possible when the body is unable to deal with the infection that plaque continues to develop and a sudden heart attack could occur.

Researchers are careful to say that not all infections result in hardening of the arteries and that other factors, such as free radicals, high blood pressure and diabetes also cause injuries to the arterial wall and encourage plaque formation. However, anything that will compromise immunity such as poor diet, stress, or serious illness may also make the body vulnerable to chronic infection and cause hardening of the arteries.

> *One out of every two people you know will die from heart disease or a stroke.*

While antibiotics are effective against bacterial infections, infections caused by viruses remain untouched. However, both bacteria and viruses can be destroyed by the medium-chain fatty acids (MCFA) found in coconut oil. MCFA are highly potent germ fighters and can kill dozens of disease-causing organisms. Coconut oil can not only protect you from germs that cause herpes, ulcers and lung infections but also from heart disease and stroke.

DID YOU KNOW? In Sri Lanka where coconut oil has been a primary dietary fat, the death rate from heart disease is the lowest in the world. Sadly, as more polyunsaturated fats have replaced coconut oil, heart disease rates are rising sharply. These so-called "heart-friendly" oils are clearly not good for the heart at all. Researchers who have seen this trend are encouraging people in India to switch back to coconut oil to reduce their heart disease risk.

Action Step: Replace vegetable oil with coconut oil to protect your heart.

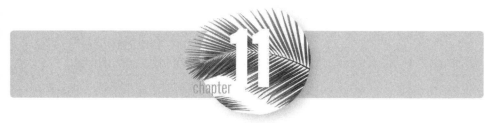

chapter **11**

Beautiful Skin

A study conducted in 2008 at the Skin and Cancer Foundation in the Philippines compared virgin coconut oil and virgin olive oil in moisturizing dryness and removing bacteria from colonized atopic dermatitis.

The study, a double-blind controlled trial, found that coconut oil was more effective than olive oil in killing bacteria, mostly because of its lauric acid content.

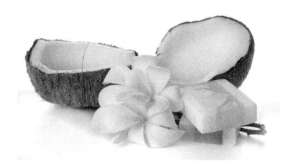

The Alternative Daily

A 2009 study at the Division of Dermatology, Department of Medicine, University of California, San Diego, looked at the antimicrobial properties of lauric acid and its potential to heal acne. The results were favorable for using lauric acid in place of antibiotics for treatment of acne.

Coconut oil helps to clear away dead skin cells and can also be combined with coconut crystals, sea salt or other natural exfoliating substances to make a very useful facial scrub that leaves the skin feeling soft and clean. No need to spend money on special products when you can use coconut oil. A simple scrub can be made by mixing one cup of coconut crystals with 1/2 cup of organic coconut oil.

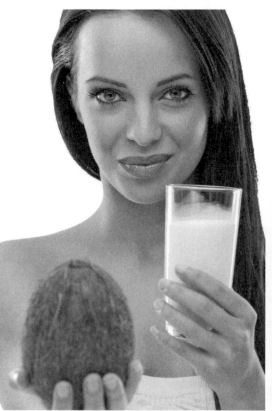

People living in the tropics have beautiful, wrinkle-free skin and this is due, in part, to their use of coconut oil. This medium-chain fatty acid protects and heals the skin at the same time. Coconut oil is also an effective sunscreen, blocking out 20 percent of harmful rays.

Coconut oil puts nutrients back into your skin, as opposed to other oils and commercial products that suffocate the skin and provide no nutritional benefits. If you want to use coconut oil as a moisturizer, be sure to start with a very small amount. If you put too much on your skin, it will not be able to drink it all in. A little goes a long way and this makes it an extremely economical choice for a moisturizer.

Coconut oil is safe for children of all ages, including babies, and can help heal up a mean diaper rash in no time.

Vitamin D Helps Fight against Skin Cancer

If you have ever known a Filipino person, you know they likely have a lovely, youthful complexion and soft, wrinkle-free skin, despite the fact that they live in a climate that exposes them to the sun's hot rays all year round. Skin cancer is virtually unheard of in the Philippines, where coconut oil is the main dietary oil used and the main ingredient in their skin care products.

Tropical Skin Exfoliant: Mix 2 parts organic brown sugar and 1 part organic extra virgin coconut oil.

The Alternative Daily

In the United States, we run scared from the sun, covering every square inch of exposed skin with lotions, lathers and sprays thinking that we are doing the right thing to protect ourselves from the damaging rays of the scorching sun. We are constantly bombarded with reasons why we need to use sunscreen, which blocks out the skin's ability to absorb vitamin D. Interestingly enough, vitamin D has been proven to prevent cancer.

Coconut oil is the main reason why people in the tropics can be in the sun and not experience skin cancer. Its healing antioxidant powers protect the skin from free radical damage. In addition, using coconut oil on the skin helps our bodies absorb other nutrients more effectively, such as vitamin E, which is another skin protecting antioxidant.

Now, don't think that you can be crazy and lay in the sun all day, even with coconut oil on your skin. You still have to be smart about the sun. Stay clear of the sun during the hottest time of the day between noon and 3 p.m., if possible. Vitamin D production is important, but it only takes a little while per day in the sun to get what you need.

The evidence that commercial sunscreen does more harm than good is very compelling. Sunscreen contains dangerous chemicals that keep the skin from breathing, and blocks beneficial sun rays. The false security that this multi-million dollar business provides is horrifying. Why not switch to an all-natural, safe and effective alternative?

Action Step: Daily use of organic, virgin coconut oil as a skin moisturizer and skin repairer may help your skin stay healthy and beautiful.

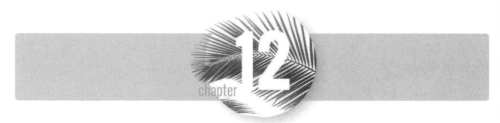

Starving Cancer Cells

Conventional cancer treatment involves chemotherapy and radiation. However, chemotherapy is a cytotoxic poison and radiation is extremely hard on the body. More often, the treatment ends up killing the patient. According to Dr. Seyfried, PhD, one of the leaders in treating cancer nutritionally, "this can no longer be accepted as the best we can do." He goes on to say, "the reason why we have so few people surviving is because of the standard of care. It has to be changed, if it's not changed, there will be no major progress. Period."

Dr. Dominic D'Agostino and a team of researchers from the University of South Florida study metabolic therapy. They discovered that when lab animals were fed a diet free of carbs, they were able to survive highly aggressive metastatic cancer much better than those treated with chemotherapy. How does this work?

The cells in the body are fueled by glucose, including cancer cells. However, cancer cells do not have the same metabolic flexibility as normal cells and can not use ketone bodies for fuel.

When you change your diet to what is known as a "fat-adapted" diet, your body uses fat for fuel rather than carbs. When you replace all carbs for healthy fats you basically starve the cancer cells as they no longer have glucose to thrive on. Once cancer cells have no fuel, you can give other preventative measures a chance to work.

Cancer Cell Starvation Diet

The first step to adopting a cancer cell starvation diet is to cut out all processed foods and drinks. These foods are loaded with sugar and contain trans fats. Adopting a whole foods, grain-free diet is essential. Another key ingredient to killing cancer cells is to replace the unhealthy carbs with healthy fat and eat only organic, pastured protein. Here are some options for healthy fats:

- ⬤ Coconuts and coconut oil
- ⬤ Olives and olive oil

The Alternative Daily

- Grass-fed butter

- Organic raw nuts, especially macadamia nuts

- Organic pastured egg yolks

- Pastured meats

- Avocados

Of course, in addition to adopting a diet high in healthy fat and low in processed carbs, the following are recommended:

- Reduce stress

- Exercise

- Get enough sleep

- Address vitamin D deficiency

Note: This type of diet is not just for those suffering from cancer, but for anyone seeking optimal health.

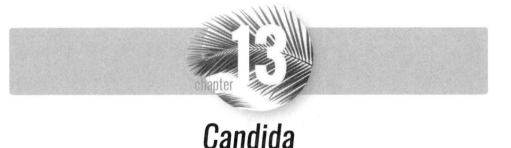

Candida

You have probably heard the word candida but may not be exactly sure about what it is. Candida is a fungus, which is actually a form of yeast. Everyone has a small amount of yeast living in their mouth and intestines. It serves an important role when it comes to digestion and nutrient absorption, but when it overpopulates, it actually breaks down the walls of the intestines and seeps into the bloodstream, where it releases toxins. This leakage can cause a number of health conditions ranging from digestive disturbances to depression.

In countries where coconuts are a dietary staple, the occurrences of

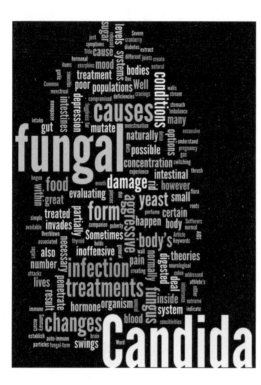

candida are quite low despite the fact that their residents live in regions that typically promote candida overgrowth. It is believed that the unique combination of healthy fatty acids, which contain antifungal, antiviral and antibacterial properties, help to balance intestinal flora and protect the body from yeast overgrowth.

Healthy Bacteria Is Good

We all have a certain amount of healthy gut bacteria which works to keep yeast levels healthy. However, many things can lead to candida getting out of control and overpowering the healthy bacteria. The good news is, we have control over most, if not all, of the factors contributing to it.

Eating a diet loaded with refined sugar and carbohydrates, a diet rich in sugar or a diet laden with foods that convert to sugar, like processed foods made with refined grains and alcohol, all encourage yeast growth. The sugar creates a perfect environment for the yeast to thrive and quickly multiply.

How Candida Gets Out of Control

1. **Taking oral contraceptives**—Taking a birth control pill causes an upset in hormones, which disrupts the good bacteria in the gut.

2. **Living a very high-stress life**—When you are stressed, the body releases cortisol, a hormone that depresses your immune system and increases blood sugar. The yeast feeds on the increased sugar and the immune system is too weak to stop it, and growth gets out of hand. In addition, if you remain stressed for a long period of time, your adrenal glands become ineffective and your immune system can be further compromised.

3. **Antibiotics**—While antibiotics effectively kill the harmful bacteria that make you sick, they also kill the friendly bacteria in your digestive system. This leaves you defenseless to fungus and yeast, which can quickly take over your gut.

How Do I Know if I Have a Yeast Problem?

Many people have a variety of candida symptoms but fail to connect the dots. Here are just a few of the warning signs to watch out for:

- Fungal infections on skin or nails— athlete's foot or toenail fungus

- Fatigue or fibromyalgia

- Constipation, bloating or diarrhea

- Bad breath

- Dry mouth

- Joint pain

- Numbness

- Hair loss

- Headaches

- PMS

- Heartburn

- Burning eyes

- Lack of impulse control

- Hyperactivity

- Poor concentration, brain fog, lack of focus, ADD, ADHD

- Autoimmune disease such as rheumatoid arthritis, lupus, ulcerative colitis or multiple sclerosis

- Mood swings, anxiety or depression

- Strong cravings for sugar or refined carbohydrates

- Skin conditions such as eczema, psoriasis, rashes or hives

- Seasonal allergies or itchy ears

- Urinary tract infections, vaginal or rectal itching

Top Eight Foods that Encourage Yeast Overgrowth

The following foods can create and make an already existing yeast problem much worse:

- Breads
- Pizza
- Fast food
- Dairy
- Soda
- Juice
- Alcohol
- Fruit

Spit Test for Yeast

Yeah, we know, it sounds a little gross, but a spit test offers a really good analysis of what is going on inside your body and may give you a sign that yeast is a problem. The best time to take this test is as soon as you wake up in the morning, before you even get out of bed.

Here is how you do it:

1. Gather as much spit as possible in your mouth.

2. Spit into a clear glass with room temperature filtered water.

3. Watch carefully.

4. The saliva will float at first - watch to see if there are thin projections extending downward into the water after 15 minutes or so. They may look like hairs or strings. If this happens you may have a candida overgrowth problem.

5. If your saliva is very cloudy and sinks to the bottom within a few minutes or parts of the saliva slowly sink, yeast overgrowth is a possibility. The particles are yeast colonies which band together.

6. If your spit is still floating after about an hour, it is likely that your yeast is under control.

The Alternative Daily

I Have Yeast, What Now?

According to the National Candida Center, if you have symptoms and your spit test is positive for yeast, it is a pretty good indication that you have a candida overgrowth problem. The first step in addressing the problem is to adjust your diet.

Eliminate all processed foods and sugar and begin eating only wholesome, organic foods if possible. The following foods also help the body heal from the assault of candida overgrowth and encourage the proliferation of healthy bacteria:

Coconut Oil—The strong antifungal, antiviral and antibacterial properties mentioned above will kill the bad bacteria, promote healthy bacterial growth and support proper immune system functioning.

Garlic—Garlic also has strong antifungal properties and will destroy unfriendly bacteria while encouraging the growth of good bacteria. It detoxifies and encourages healthy liver and colon functioning. Use garlic liberally to jazz up your food or chew freely on 2–3 cloves per day. Note: raw garlic is far superior in its efficacy.

Seaweed—It may not be too appealing to look at, but seaweed is a highly nutrient-dense food that can fight against yeast overgrowth. Many times, persons with yeast suffer from hypothyroidism.

Seaweed is rich in iodine, which helps balance the thyroid gland. In addition, seaweed is a detoxifier and helps to flush toxins out of the body while cleaning the digestive system. Eat fresh seaweed or take high quality kelp supplements for best results.

Pumpkin Seeds—These tiny seeds are packed with omega-3 fatty acids, which have antiviral and antifungal properties. They help to reduce the inflammation caused by yeast, and also fight depression. Add pumpkin seeds to your cereal and salads, or even eat them on their own as a tasty snack.

Ginger—Ginger is a powerful detoxifier that increases circulation and flushes toxins out of the liver while supporting the immune system. It helps reduce intestinal gas and soothes inflammation from yeast overgrowth. Make ginger tea by grating a 1-inch piece of ginger root and adding it to 2 cups of boiling water and a fresh slice of lemon.

Once you get your diet under control and introduce foods that fight the bad bacteria, you can consider taking a high-quality probiotic or eating a few fermented foods daily to keep your healthy bacteria count in good order.

The Alternative Daily

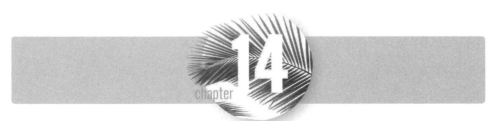

Increased Nutrient Availability

MCTs are easily absorbed in the digestive tract and also improve the rate at which other nutrients are absorbed. A Denmark study compared absorption of fat in patients who had had their colon completely or partially removed. Patients were fed a diet consisting of either long-chain fatty acids or half medium-chain fatty acids and half long-chain fatty acids. Those that were fed long-chain fatty acids alone deposited fat in their feces, as it was not absorbed in the bowel. The group that consumed the medium-chain fatty acids along with the long-chain fatty acids not only absorbed these fatty acids better, but also absorbed the long-chain fatty acids better.

Another study compared sunflower oil to coconut oil on mice and found that mice fed a diet of MCTs had reduced intestinal inflammation and reduced incidences of colitis. Many people tend to find relief from ulcerative colitis, Crohn's disease and IBS after adding coconut oil to their diet.

This page intentionally left blank.

12 Healthy Coconut Oil Recipes

Table of Contents

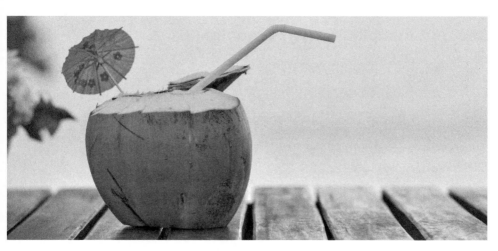

Cooking with coconut oil is easy and healthy. Use organic, extra virgin coconut oil for all of these recipes.

Breakfast Options

Blueberry Coconut Smoothie

* You can substitute any fruit for the blueberries to change this smoothie around.

- 1/2 cup organic Greek yogurt
- 2/3 cup organic coconut milk
- 1 1/2 teaspoons pure vanilla extract
- 1/2 cup frozen or fresh blueberries*
- 2 tablespoons melted coconut oil

To Make: Blend everything together but add the coconut oil in slowly while mixing. Serve with coconut flakes for a garnish.

Coconut Pumpkin Energy Smoothie

- 1/4 cup pumpkin puree
- 1 frozen banana
- 1/2 cup coconut or organic almond milk
- A dash of cinnamon
- 1 teaspoon raw honey
- 1 teaspoon chia seeds
- 1 tablespoon coconut oil, melted

To Make: Blend everything together but add the coconut oil in slowly while mixing. Serve with crushed cinnamon for a garnish.

Chocolate-Coconut Overnight Oats

- 15–16 ounces coconut or organic almond milk
- 1 cup water
- 1 cup shredded coconut
- 2 tablespoons chia seeds
- 4 tablespoons raw cacao powder
- 4 tablespoons raw honey
- 1 tablespoon coconut oil
- 1 cup gluten-free rolled oats

To Make: Mix everything but the oats together in a blender until well mixed. Pour over the oats and cover. Set in the refrigerator overnight.

Lunch/Side Options

Coconut Stir-fry Vegetables

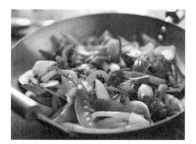

** Feel free to experiment by adding
some of your own favorite vegetables.*

- 2 tablespoons coconut oil
- Red pepper cut into small chunks
- Yellow pepper cut into small chunks
- Red onion thinly sliced
- 1 large sweet potato cut into small chunks
- 1 cup broccoli florets
- 1 clove minced garlic
- 2 cups sliced bok choy
- 1/2 cup snap peas
- 1 cup mung bean sprouts
- 2 tablespoons sesame oil
- Sea salt

To Make: Cut up all of your veggies so you are ready to stir fry. In a large skillet or a wok, heat the coconut oil over a medium heat. Add the sweet potatoes first and cook until slightly soft. Add the other ingredients and stir constantly until crisp. Add sea salt to taste and serve over brown rice.

The Alternative Daily

Cheesy Coconut Rice

- 2 organic eggs
- 2 cups cooked brown rice
- 4 tablespoons coconut oil
- 4 ounces shredded extra sharp cheddar cheese
- Sea salt

To Make: Whisk the eggs in a small bowl and set aside. Melt the coconut oil in medium sauté pan and when it is hot, add the rice and stir-fry. Move the rice to one side of the pan and pour the beaten egg into the middle. Scramble the eggs until they are almost done and mix in the rice. Add the cheese and stir until melted. Add salt to taste.

Coconut Mashed Potatoes

- 2 pounds of organic red potatoes
- 1/4 cup coconut oil
- 2 tablespoon of organic butter
- 1/2 cup organic sour cream
- 1 cup of coconut milk at room temperature
- Sea salt and fresh pepper

To Make: Wash the potatoes and steam until soft (leave the skin on). Add the oil, sour cream and butter and blend with a mixer until smooth. Add the coconut milk slowly and season with salt and pepper.

Roasted Broccoli and Cauliflower Bake

- ◆ 2 organic broccoli crowns
- ◆ 1 head organic purple cauliflower
- ◆ 3 tablespoons coconut oil
- ◆ 5 cloves crushed garlic
- ◆ 2 tablespoons fresh lemon juice

To Make: Wash the broccoli and cauliflower, chop into small chunks and place in a 9x13-inch pan. Drizzle coconut oil, lemon and garlic on top and stir. Bake for 25 minutes at 350 degrees F or until tender.

Coconut Spinach Salad

- ◆ 1 tablespoon organic tomato paste
- ◆ 1 tablespoon organic mustard
- ◆ 1 tablespoon coconut water vinegar
- ◆ 1 teaspoon organic virgin olive oil
- ◆ 1 tablespoon coconut oil, warmed
- ◆ 1/2 cup raw mozzarella cheese, grated
- ◆ 4 cups organic spinach
- ◆ 2 tablespoons organic dried unsweetened coconut

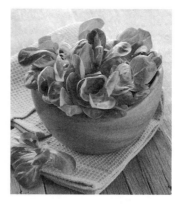

To Make: Combine all in a large bowl and serve immediately.

The Alternative Daily

Roasted Coconut Sweet Potatoes

- 7–8 cups of organic sweet potatoes
- 1/2 cup raw pecan halves
- 4 tablespoons melted coconut oil
- 4 tablespoon maple syrup
- 2 tablespoons organic coconut sugar
- 1 1/2 teaspoons cinnamon
- 1 1/2 teaspoons nutmeg
- 1/2 teaspoon sea salt
- 1 teaspoon chia seeds

To Make: Peel and cut the potatoes into 1-inch pieces. Combine all ingredients in a 9x13 pan and toss until potatoes are well coated. Bake at 400 degrees F until the potatoes are tender—stirring occasionally. When done, sprinkle with chia seeds and serve warm.

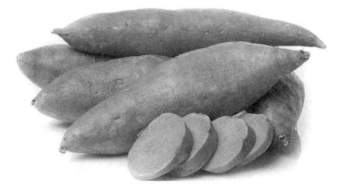

Dinner/Main Dish Options

Coconut Fried Flounder

- 4 fresh-caught flounder filets
- 1 cup organic buttermlk
- 1/3 cup coconut flour
- 1/4 cup organic cornmeal
- 1/3 cup gluten-free breadcrumbs
- Sea salt and pepper
- Cayenne pepper
- 4 tablespoons coconut oil
- Juice of 2 lemons

To Make: Soak the fish in the buttermilk and mix flour, breadcrumbs, cornmeal and spices together. Coat the fillets in the flour mixture on both sides. Heat the oil on medium heat and place the fillets in the hot skillet. Brown on one side and turn to the other—add in 2 more tablespoons of coconut

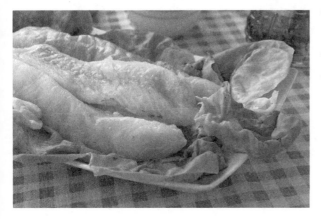

oil and remove when brown. Squeeze the fresh lemon juice over the fish and serve immediately.

The Alternative Daily

Coconut Chicken

- 1 whole organic free-range chicken cut up in small to medium pieces
- Coconut milk to cover chicken
- 2 fresh limes, juiced
- 2 cloves garlic, minced
- 1/4 cup chopped yellow onion
- Sea salt and pepper
- 1 cup coconut flour
- 1/2 cup unsweetened coconut flakes
- Tuscan seasoning
- 2 tablespoons coconut oil

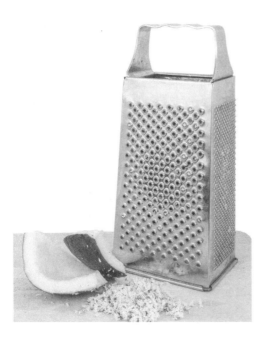

To Make: Mix together coconut milk, lime juice, garlic, onion and salt and pepper and marinate chicken for at least 2 hours. Mix coconut flour, coconut flakes and seasoning together. Cover chicken in the flour mixture and press extra coconut flakes into chicken. Place chicken in a glass pan coated in coconut oil. Drizzle melted coconut oil on top of the chicken. Bake at 350 degrees F for 45 minutes.

Coconut Sauteed Shrimp

- 3 tablespoons coconut oil
- 6 organic green onions (white parts sliced) keep green parts
- 1 tablespoon fresh minced ginger
- 2 cloves garlic
- 1/2 teaspoon ground coriander
- 1/2 teaspoon sea salt
- Juice of 1 lemon
- 1/2 teaspoon ground black pepper
- 1 pound uncooked shrimp

To Make: Melt the coconut oil in a large skillet over medium heat. Add the onions, garlic and ginger. Cook until fragrant. Add the coriander and cook for about 30 seconds. Toss in the shrimp and add salt. Cook until the shrimp are opaque, usually about 3 minutes. Stir green onion parts and cook until wilted. Season with lemon juice and pepper. Serve with a side of lemon.

This page intentionally left blank.

20 Ways to Use Coconut Oil

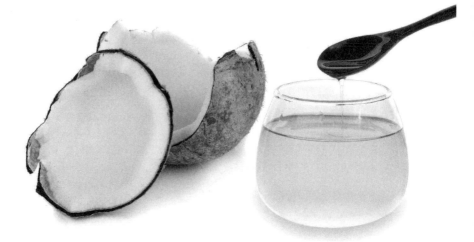

Coconut oil coffee: Add 1 tablespoon to your morning coffee for a super energy burst. Simply put it in the coffee and blend.

Cut and wound relief: The antimicrobial action of coconut oil kills bacteria and harmful microbes while promoting healing. Clean the wound thoroughly, and when dry, apply a small amount of coconut oil to the affected area.

Toothpaste: Bypass glycerin and sodium fluoride by making your own healthy toothpaste blend. Simply mix 6 tablespoons of coconut oil with 6 tablespoons of baking soda, then add 25 drops of peppermint essential oil, plus 1 teaspoon of raw stevia for a sweetener. Use as you would regular toothpaste.

Sore throat: Coconut oil contains anti-inflammatory properties that help ease irritation and promote healing of a sore throat. The antimicrobial properties also fight fungi, bacteria and even viruses. Warm a teaspoon of oil and allow it to drip coat the back of the throat. You can also make a soothing syrup that will help ease throat pain and reduce coughing. Mix 3 tablespoons of freshly squeezed lemon juice with 1/4 cup local raw honey and 2 tablespoons of coconut oil in a small saucepan and warm over a low heat. Mix the syrup in warm water or tea.

Hair conditioner: The fatty acids in coconut oil nourish hair at the roots. You can replace expensive, synthetic products with coconut oil and your hair will be silky and shiny. To condition your hair,

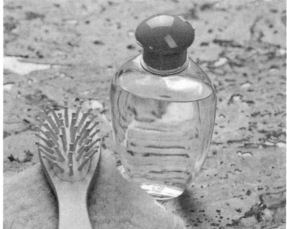

pour 1 cup of hot water into a small bowl. Add 2 teaspoons of coconut oil to the water. Allow the oil to melt and massage into damp or dry hair. Comb the oil through your hair and place a shower cap on your head. Let the coconut oil set for at least an hour or even overnight. Wash your hair twice to remove excess oil.

The Alternative Daily

Makeup remover: Conventional makeup removal products tend to dry the skin and can even promote aging. Place a small dab of coconut oil on a clean cotton pad and gently wipe away makeup. Your skin will feel fresh and moisturized.

Lip Balm: Moisten and heal dry and chapped lips with soothing coconut oil. You can make a soothing lip balm by combining 1/8 cup of coconut oil with 1/4 cup beeswax, 1/8 cup shea butter, 1 tablespoon pure vanilla extract and 1 teaspoon of sweet almond oil. Melt the ingredients over low to medium heat and pour into small containers.

Aftershave: Use a small amount of coconut oil to replenish your skin after shaving. Simply rub into skin to soothe razor burn and promote healing. Remember, a little goes a long way.

Nail fungus: When yeast becomes overgrown it can result in nail fungus. The antifungal properties of coconut oil can stop the overgrowth in its tracks. Apply a little coconut oil to the infected nail morning and night and also consume at least 1 tablespoon of coconut oil daily to improve systemic infections.

Eczema: The antibacterial and antioxidant powers in coconut oil help soothe itchy and sore skin without harsh chemicals. Apply several times a day to affected area for relief.

Season cast iron skillets: If you love your cast iron skillet you know that one of the things you must do is season it. To season, melt 1 teaspoon of oil in the pan and then use a paper towel to spread a thin layer of oil all over your pan, top, bottom and handle. Heat the oven to 400 degrees F and place your pan upside down on a rack. Be sure to line the bottom of your oven in foil to catch any oil drips. Bake your pan for one hour and allow it to cool.

Deodorant: Coconut oil contains lauric acid which fights odor. You may think that coconut oil would stain your clothes, however, a light layer applied daily will not stain. To make your own deodorant, mix 1/4 cup baking soda, 1/4 cup arrowroot powder, 1/3 cup of coconut oil, 5 drops of orange essential oil and 4 drops of tea tree essential oil. Mix everything together well and put in a small container.

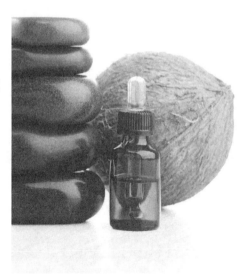

Insect repellant: To keep bugs away and condition your skin at the same time, mix equal parts of coconut and neem oil together. Apply a light layer before going outdoors.

Nail and cuticle growth enhancer: The nutrients in coconut oil strengthen cuticles and nails. Applying a light layer of oil once or twice a week will keep your nails and cuticles strong and fight any cuticle infections and fungus that may be on your nails. Healthy nails will grow more quickly than unhealthy nails.

Sticker remover: To make your own non-toxic version, mix equal parts of coconut oil and baking soda. Store in an airtight container.

Age spots: The antioxidants in coconut oil will not only help protect you from age spots, but also help to fade spots you already have. Apply a few drops of coconut oil to clean skin and massage the spots using upwards strokes. To help prevent age spots from forming, apply some coconut oil to your skin immediately after coming out of the sun.

Diaper rash: Coconut oil is a safe and effective way to protect your baby's soft bottom. Use for diaper rash as well as cradle cap. Remember, a little goes a long way. Keep a small jar in your diaper bag and on your changing station.

Canker sores: Daily oil pulling with coconut oil will keep canker sores at bay. If you happen to get a canker sore, simply consume 1 tablespoon of coconut oil 3 times a day in warm water or on its own. The antibacterial properties in the oil will go to work to fight bacteria and heal the skin inside your mouth.

Popcorn: Microwave popcorn contains some dangerous ingredients, mostly in the bag and in the oil. Go back to cooking popcorn on the stove, the old-fashioned way using coconut oil. Not only will you benefit from the nutritional value of the oil but your popcorn will have a light, tropical taste.

Moisturize leather: Don't buy expensive leather moisturizer when you can use a little bit of coconut oil on a soft cloth. After cleaning your leather, use a little bit of coconut oil to moisturize any leather product.

The Alternative Daily

Summing It All Up

Now that you have read this book, we hope you have a new-found understanding and appreciation for coconut oil. Coconuts and the oil that they produce are truly a gift from nature that can easily help create a strong foundation for a healthy lifestyle.

Coconut oil is safe, versatile and does not produce any negative side effects or have any contradictions with other medicinal therapies. Both complementary and mainstream medicine are beginning to meet on level ground about coconut oil, and it is not uncommon these days for a general health practitioner to recommend its use for a number of conditions or as a general health supplement.

If you are still using unhealthy oils to cook with, now is the best time to make the switch to coconut oil. Don't forget that coconut oil is also easily incorporated into your beauty regimen as well as your home first-aid kit. Its potent medicinal and dietary compounds make it a useful and rewarding household staple.

To Your Health!

Sources

Assuncao, M.L. (2009). Effects of dietary coconut oil on the biochemical and anthropometric profiles of women presenting abdominal obesity. *Lipids*, 44 (7), 593-601. doi: 10.1007/s11745-009-3306-6

Caprylic Acid: The Extraordinary Saturated Fatty Acid that Heals Rather than Harms. (2007). *The Healthier Life*. Retrieved from http://www.thehealthierlife.co.uk/natural-health-articles/nutrition/caprylic-acid-healing-properties-00348/

DeBakey, M. (1964). Serum Cholesterol Values in Patients Treated Surgically for Atherosclerosis. *JAMA*, 189, 655-659. Retrieved from http://www.ncbi.nlm.nih.gov/pubmed/14172263

Fife, B. (2004). *The Coconut Oil Miracle: Fourth Revised Edition*. New York: Avery Publishing Group.

Gura, T. (1998). Infections: a cause of artery-clogging plaques? Science, 281 (5373), 35-37. Retrieved from http://www.ncbi.nlm.nih.gov/pubmed/9679016

Heini, A.F., & Weinsier, R.L. (1996). Divergent trends in obesity and fat intake patterns: the American paradox. *The American Journal of Medicine*, 102 (3), 259-264. http://dx.doi.org/10.1016/S0002-9343(96)00456-1

The Alternative Daily

Hoshimoto, A. et al. (2002) Caprylic acid and medium-chain triglycerides inhibit IL-8 gene transcription in Caco-2 cells: comparison with the potent histone deacetylase inhibitor trichostatin A. *British Journal of Pharmacology,* 136 (2), 280-286. doi: 10.1038/sj.bjp.0704719

Kaunitz, H. (1986). Medium chain triglycerides (MCT) in aging and arteriosclerosis. *Journal of Environmental Pathology, Toxicology, and Oncology,* 6 (3-4), 115-121. Retrieved from http://www.ncbi.nlm.nih.gov/pubmed/3519928

Kim, B.H. (2010). The effects of high dietary lard on hypertension development in spontaneously hypertensive rats. *Journal of Medicinal Food,* 13 (5), 1263-1272. doi: 10.1089/jmf.2010.1015

Krishna, G. (2010). *Coconut Oil: Chemistry, Production and Its Applications: A Review. Indian Coconut Journal.* Retrieved from http://coconutboard.nic.in/English-Article-Gopalakrishna-CFTRI.pdf

Lackland, D.T. (1990). The need for accurate nutrition survey methodology: the South Carolina experience. *Journal of Nutrition,* 120 (11), 1433-1466. Retrieved from http://www.ncbi.nlm.nih.gov/pubmed/2243282

Liau, K.M. (2011). An Open-Label Pilot Study to Assess the Efficacy and Safety of Virgin Coconut Oil in Reducing Visceral Adiposity. ISRN Pharmacology, 949686. doi: 10.5402/2011/949686

Marina, A.M. (2009). Antioxidant capacity and phenolic acids of virgin coconut oil. *International Journal of Food Sciences and Nutrition,* 60, 114-123. doi: 10.1080/09637480802549127

Medical Economics, et al. (2001). The PDR Guide to Nutritional Supplements. *Physician's Desk Reference.* New York: Thomson PDR

Nevin, K.G. (2010). Effect of topical application of virgin coconut oil on skin components and antioxidant status during dermal wound healing in young rats. *Skin Pharmacology and Physiology,* 23 (6), 290-297. doi: 10.1159/000313516

McClernon, F.J. (2007). The effects of a low-carbohydrate ketogenic diet and a low-fat diet on mood, hunger, and other self-reported symptoms. *Obesity (Silver Spring), 15 (1)*, 182-187. Retrieved from http://www.ncbi.nlm.nih.gov/pubmed/17228046

Nakatsuji, T. (2009). Antimicrobial property of lauric acid against Propionibacterium acnes: its therapeutic potential for inflammatory acne vulgaris. *The Journal of Investigative Dermatology,* 129 (10), 2480-2488. doi: 10.1038/jid.2009.93

National Candida Center http://www.NationalCandidaCenter.com

Rahman, H. (2000). *The Chemistry of Coconut Oil,* Universiti Brunei Darussalam. Retrieved from http://fos.ubd.edu.bn/sites/default/files/2000-Paper2.pdf

Shilhavy, B. & Shilhavy, M. http://CoconutOil.com

Sircar, S. (1998). Choice of cooking oils -- myths and realities. *Journal of the Indian Medical Association,* 96 (10), 304-307. Retrieved from http://www.ncbi.nlm.nih.gov/pubmed/10063298

St. Onge, M.P. (2003). Greater rise in fat oxidation with medium-chain triglyceride consumption relative to long-chain triglyceride is associated with lower initial body weight and greater loss of subcutaneous adipose tissue. *International Journal of Obesity and Related Metabolic Disorders*, 27 (12), 1565-1571. Retrieved from http://www.ncbi.nlm.nih.gov/pubmed/12975635

St. Onge, M.P. (2003). Medium-chain triglycerides increase energy expenditure and decrease adiposity in overweight men. *Obesity Research*, 11 (3), 395-402. Retrieved from http://www.ncbi.nlm.nih.gov/pubmed/12634436

Stubbs, R.J. (1996). Covert manipulation of the ratio of medium- to long-chain triglycerides in isoenergetically dense diets: effect on food intake in ad libitum feeding men. International J*ournal of Obesity and Related Metabolic Disorders, 20 (5)*, 435-444. Retrieved from http://www.ncbi.nlm.nih.gov/pubmed/8696422

Van Wymelbeke, V. (1998). Influence of medium-chain and long-chain triacylglycerols on the control of food intake in men. *The American Journal of Clinical Nutrition, 68 (2)*, 226-234. Retrieved from http://www.ncbi.nlm.nih.gov/pubmed/9701177

Verallo-Rowell, V.M. (2008). Novel antibacterial and emollient effects of coconut and virgin olive oils in adult atopic dermatitis. *Dermatitis, 19 (6),* 308-315. Retrieved from http://www.ncbi.nlm.nih.gov/pubmed/19134433